This book belongs to	
Name	
Address	
Phone	
Email	

ISBN 978-0-244-02778-0

T.L Crofts
250 Gumma Road, Gumma
New South Wales, Australia, 2447

MENTAL HEALTH

Daily

SYMPTOM TRACKER

T.L CROFTS

Day: Date: /   /20

Physical	Morn	After	Eve	12am+
headache				
nausea				
pain				
menstrual				
fatigue				

Emotional	Morn	After	Eve	12am+
anxious				
calm				
panic				
irritable				
overwhelmed				
depressed				
manic				
excited				
content				

Mental	Morn	After	Eve	12am+
hopeless				
hopeful				
distracted				
focused				
bored				
ideas				
dissociated				
aware				

Weather:

Meds		Energy Levels	
am		5 - high	
pm		4	
		3	
Hygiene		2	
brush teeth		1 - low	
shower			
change clothes		**Food**	
Intake			
caffeine			
alcohol			
water			
TV			
social media			
time outside		**Creative Space**	
Sleep Hours			
dreamy			
restless			
light			
deep			
terror			

Notes - Wins

Day: Date: /   /20

Physical	Morn	After	Eve	12am+
headache				
nausea				
pain				
menstrual				
fatigue				

Emotional	Morn	After	Eve	12am+
anxious				
calm				
panic				
irritable				
overwhelmed				
depressed				
manic				
excited				
content				

Mental	Morn	After	Eve	12am+
hopeless				
hopeful				
distracted				
focused				
bored				
ideas				
dissociated				
aware				

Weather:

Meds		Energy Levels	
am		5 - high	
pm		4	
		3	
Hygiene		2	
brush teeth		1 - low	
shower			
change clothes		**Food**	
Intake			
caffeine			
alcohol			
water			
TV			
social media			
time outside		**Creative Space**	
Sleep Hours			
dreamy			
restless			
light			
deep			
terror			

Notes - Wins

Day: Date: /   /20

Physical	Morn	After	Eve	12am+
headache				
nausea				
pain				
menstrual				
fatigue				
Emotional	**Morn**	**After**	**Eve**	**12am+**
anxious				
calm				
panic				
irritable				
overwhelmed				
depressed				
manic				
excited				
content				
Mental	**Morn**	**After**	**Eve**	**12am+**
hopeless				
hopeful				
distracted				
focused				
bored				
ideas				
dissociated				
aware				

Weather:

Meds		Energy Levels	
am		5 - high	
pm		4	
		3	
Hygiene		2	
brush teeth		1 - low	
shower			
change clothes		**Food**	
Intake			
caffeine			
alcohol			
water			
TV			
social media			
time outside		**Creative Space**	
Sleep Hours			
dreamy			
restless			
light			
deep			
terror			

Notes - Wins

Day: Date: /   /20

Physical	Morn	After	Eve	12am+
headache				
nausea				
pain				
menstrual				
fatigue				

Emotional	Morn	After	Eve	12am+
anxious				
calm				
panic				
irritable				
overwhelmed				
depressed				
manic				
excited				
content				

Mental	Morn	After	Eve	12am+
hopeless				
hopeful				
distracted				
focused				
bored				
ideas				
dissociated				
aware				

Weather:

Meds		Energy Levels	
am		5 - high	
pm		4	
		3	
Hygiene		2	
brush teeth		1 - low	
shower			
change clothes		**Food**	
Intake			
caffeine			
alcohol			
water			
TV			
social media			
time outside		**Creative Space**	
Sleep Hours			
dreamy			
restless			
light			
deep			
terror			

Notes - Wins

Day: Date: /   /20

Physical	Morn	After	Eve	12am+
headache				
nausea				
pain				
menstrual				
fatigue				

Emotional	Morn	After	Eve	12am+
anxious				
calm				
panic				
irritable				
overwhelmed				
depressed				
manic				
excited				
content				

Mental	Morn	After	Eve	12am+
hopeless				
hopeful				
distracted				
focused				
bored				
ideas				
dissociated				
aware				

Weather:

Meds		Energy Levels	
am		5 - high	
pm		4	
		3	
Hygiene		2	
brush teeth		1 - low	
shower			
change clothes		**Food**	
Intake			
caffeine			
alcohol			
water			
TV			
social media			
time outside		**Creative Space**	
Sleep Hours			
dreamy			
restless			
light			
deep			
terror			

Notes - Wins

Day: Date: /   /20

Physical	Morn	After	Eve	12am+
headache				
nausea				
pain				
menstrual				
fatigue				

Emotional	Morn	After	Eve	12am+
anxious				
calm				
panic				
irritable				
overwhelmed				
depressed				
manic				
excited				
content				

Mental	Morn	After	Eve	12am+
hopeless				
hopeful				
distracted				
focused				
bored				
ideas				
dissociated				
aware				

Weather:

Meds		Energy Levels	
am		5 - high	
pm		4	
		3	
Hygiene		2	
brush teeth		1 - low	
shower			
change clothes		**Food**	
Intake			
caffeine			
alcohol			
water			
TV			
social media			
time outside		**Creative Space**	
Sleep Hours			
dreamy			
restless			
light			
deep			
terror			

Notes - Wins

Day: Date: /   /20

Physical	Morn	After	Eve	12am+
headache				
nausea				
pain				
menstrual				
fatigue				

Emotional	Morn	After	Eve	12am+
anxious				
calm				
panic				
irritable				
overwhelmed				
depressed				
manic				
excited				
content				

Mental	Morn	After	Eve	12am+
hopeless				
hopeful				
distracted				
focused				
bored				
ideas				
dissociated				
aware				

Weather:

Meds		Energy Levels	
am		5 - high	
pm		4	
		3	
Hygiene		2	
brush teeth		1 - low	
shower			
change clothes		**Food**	
Intake			
caffeine			
alcohol			
water			
TV			
social media			
time outside		**Creative Space**	
Sleep Hours			
dreamy			
restless			
light			
deep			
terror			

Notes - Wins

Notes

Creative Space

Day: Date: /   /20

Physical	Morn	After	Eve	12am+
headache				
nausea				
pain				
menstrual				
fatigue				

Emotional	Morn	After	Eve	12am+
anxious				
calm				
panic				
irritable				
overwhelmed				
depressed				
manic				
excited				
content				

Mental	Morn	After	Eve	12am+
hopeless				
hopeful				
distracted				
focused				
bored				
ideas				
dissociated				
aware				

Weather:

Meds		Energy Levels	
am		5 - high	
pm		4	
		3	
Hygiene		2	
brush teeth		1 - low	
shower			
change clothes		**Food**	
Intake			
caffeine			
alcohol			
water			
TV			
social media			
time outside		**Creative Space**	
Sleep Hours			
dreamy			
restless			
light			
deep			
terror			

Notes - Wins

Day: Date: /   /20

Physical	Morn	After	Eve	12am+
headache				
nausea				
pain				
menstrual				
fatigue				

Emotional	Morn	After	Eve	12am+
anxious				
calm				
panic				
irritable				
overwhelmed				
depressed				
manic				
excited				
content				

Mental	Morn	After	Eve	12am+
hopeless				
hopeful				
distracted				
focused				
bored				
ideas				
dissociated				
aware				

Weather:

Meds		Energy Levels	
am		5 - high	
pm		4	
		3	
Hygiene		2	
brush teeth		1 - low	
shower			
change clothes		**Food**	
Intake			
caffeine			
alcohol			
water			
TV			
social media			
time outside		**Creative Space**	
Sleep Hours			
dreamy			
restless			
light			
deep			
terror			

Notes - Wins

Day: Date: /   /20

Physical	Morn	After	Eve	12am+
headache				
nausea				
pain				
menstrual				
fatigue				

Emotional	Morn	After	Eve	12am+
anxious				
calm				
panic				
irritable				
overwhelmed				
depressed				
manic				
excited				
content				

Mental	Morn	After	Eve	12am+
hopeless				
hopeful				
distracted				
focused				
bored				
ideas				
dissociated				
aware				

Weather:

Meds		Energy Levels	
am		5 - high	
pm		4	
		3	
Hygiene		2	
brush teeth		1 - low	
shower			
change clothes		**Food**	
Intake			
caffeine			
alcohol			
water			
TV			
social media			
time outside		**Creative Space**	
Sleep Hours			
dreamy			
restless			
light			
deep			
terror			

Notes - Wins

Day: Date: /   /20

Physical	Morn	After	Eve	12am+
headache				
nausea				
pain				
menstrual				
fatigue				

Emotional	Morn	After	Eve	12am+
anxious				
calm				
panic				
irritable				
overwhelmed				
depressed				
manic				
excited				
content				

Mental	Morn	After	Eve	12am+
hopeless				
hopeful				
distracted				
focused				
bored				
ideas				
dissociated				
aware				

Weather:

Meds		Energy Levels	
am		5 - high	
pm		4	
		3	
Hygiene		2	
brush teeth		1 - low	
shower			
change clothes		**Food**	
Intake			
caffeine			
alcohol			
water			
TV			
social media			
time outside		**Creative Space**	
Sleep Hours			
dreamy			
restless			
light			
deep			
terror			

Notes - Wins

Day: Date: /   /20

Physical	Morn	After	Eve	12am+
headache				
nausea				
pain				
menstrual				
fatigue				

Emotional	Morn	After	Eve	12am+
anxious				
calm				
panic				
irritable				
overwhelmed				
depressed				
manic				
excited				
content				

Mental	Morn	After	Eve	12am+
hopeless				
hopeful				
distracted				
focused				
bored				
ideas				
dissociated				
aware				

Weather:

Meds		Energy Levels	
am		5 - high	
pm		4	
		3	
Hygiene		2	
brush teeth		1 - low	
shower			
change clothes		**Food**	
Intake			
caffeine			
alcohol			
water			
TV			
social media			
time outside		**Creative Space**	
Sleep Hours			
dreamy			
restless			
light			
deep			
terror			

Notes - Wins

Day: Date: /   /20

Physical	Morn	After	Eve	12am+
headache				
nausea				
pain				
menstrual				
fatigue				

Emotional	Morn	After	Eve	12am+
anxious				
calm				
panic				
irritable				
overwhelmed				
depressed				
manic				
excited				
content				

Mental	Morn	After	Eve	12am+
hopeless				
hopeful				
distracted				
focused				
bored				
ideas				
dissociated				
aware				

Weather:

Meds		Energy Levels	
am		5 - high	
pm		4	
		3	
Hygiene		2	
brush teeth		1 - low	
shower			
change clothes		**Food**	
Intake			
caffeine			
alcohol			
water			
TV			
social media			
time outside		**Creative Space**	
Sleep Hours			
dreamy			
restless			
light			
deep			
terror			

Notes - Wins

Day: Date: /   /20

Physical	Morn	After	Eve	12am+
headache				
nausea				
pain				
menstrual				
fatigue				

Emotional	Morn	After	Eve	12am+
anxious				
calm				
panic				
irritable				
overwhelmed				
depressed				
manic				
excited				
content				

Mental	Morn	After	Eve	12am+
hopeless				
hopeful				
distracted				
focused				
bored				
ideas				
dissociated				
aware				

Weather:

Meds		Energy Levels	
am		5 - high	
pm		4	
		3	
Hygiene		2	
brush teeth		1 - low	
shower			
change clothes		**Food**	
Intake			
caffeine			
alcohol			
water			
TV			
social media			
time outside		**Creative Space**	
Sleep Hours			
dreamy			
restless			
light			
deep			
terror			

Notes - Wins

Notes

Day: Date: /   /20

Physical	Morn	After	Eve	12am+
headache				
nausea				
pain				
menstrual				
fatigue				

Emotional	Morn	After	Eve	12am+
anxious				
calm				
panic				
irritable				
overwhelmed				
depressed				
manic				
excited				
content				

Mental	Morn	After	Eve	12am+
hopeless				
hopeful				
distracted				
focused				
bored				
ideas				
dissociated				
aware				

Weather:

Meds		Energy Levels	
am		5 - high	
pm		4	
		3	
Hygiene		2	
brush teeth		1 - low	
shower			
change clothes		**Food**	
Intake			
caffeine			
alcohol			
water			
TV			
social media			
time outside		**Creative Space**	
Sleep Hours			
dreamy			
restless			
light			
deep			
terror			

Notes - Wins

Day: Date: /   /20

Physical	Morn	After	Eve	12am+
headache				
nausea				
pain				
menstrual				
fatigue				

Emotional	Morn	After	Eve	12am+
anxious				
calm				
panic				
irritable				
overwhelmed				
depressed				
manic				
excited				
content				

Mental	Morn	After	Eve	12am+
hopeless				
hopeful				
distracted				
focused				
bored				
ideas				
dissociated				
aware				

Weather:

Meds		Energy Levels	
am		5 - high	
pm		4	
		3	
Hygiene		2	
brush teeth		1 - low	
shower			
change clothes		**Food**	
Intake			
caffeine			
alcohol			
water			
TV			
social media			
time outside		**Creative Space**	
Sleep Hours			
dreamy			
restless			
light			
deep			
terror			

Notes - Wins

Day: Date: /   /20

Physical	Morn	After	Eve	12am+
headache				
nausea				
pain				
menstrual				
fatigue				

Emotional	Morn	After	Eve	12am+
anxious				
calm				
panic				
irritable				
overwhelmed				
depressed				
manic				
excited				
content				

Mental	Morn	After	Eve	12am+
hopeless				
hopeful				
distracted				
focused				
bored				
ideas				
dissociated				
aware				

Weather:

Meds		Energy Levels	
am		5 - high	
pm		4	
		3	
Hygiene		2	
brush teeth		1 - low	
shower			
change clothes		**Food**	
Intake			
caffeine			
alcohol			
water			
TV			
social media			
time outside		**Creative Space**	
Sleep Hours			
dreamy			
restless			
light			
deep			
terror			

Notes - Wins

Day: Date: / /20

Physical	Morn	After	Eve	12am+
headache				
nausea				
pain				
menstrual				
fatigue				

Emotional	Morn	After	Eve	12am+
anxious				
calm				
panic				
irritable				
overwhelmed				
depressed				
manic				
excited				
content				

Mental	Morn	After	Eve	12am+
hopeless				
hopeful				
distracted				
focused				
bored				
ideas				
dissociated				
aware				

Weather:

Meds		Energy Levels	
am		5 - high	
pm		4	
		3	
Hygiene		2	
brush teeth		1 - low	
shower			
change clothes		**Food**	
Intake			
caffeine			
alcohol			
water			
TV			
social media			
time outside		**Creative Space**	
Sleep Hours			
dreamy			
restless			
light			
deep			
terror			

Notes - Wins

Day: Date: /   /20

Physical	Morn	After	Eve	12am+
headache				
nausea				
pain				
menstrual				
fatigue				

Emotional	Morn	After	Eve	12am+
anxious				
calm				
panic				
irritable				
overwhelmed				
depressed				
manic				
excited				
content				

Mental	Morn	After	Eve	12am+
hopeless				
hopeful				
distracted				
focused				
bored				
ideas				
dissociated				
aware				

Weather:

Meds		Energy Levels	
am		5 - high	
pm		4	
		3	
Hygiene		2	
brush teeth		1 - low	
shower			
change clothes		**Food**	
Intake			
caffeine			
alcohol			
water			
TV			
social media			
time outside		**Creative Space**	
Sleep Hours			
dreamy			
restless			
light			
deep			
terror			

Notes - Wins

Day: _____   Date: /   /20

Physical	Morn	After	Eve	12am+
headache				
nausea				
pain				
menstrual				
fatigue				

Emotional	Morn	After	Eve	12am+
anxious				
calm				
panic				
irritable				
overwhelmed				
depressed				
manic				
excited				
content				

Mental	Morn	After	Eve	12am+
hopeless				
hopeful				
distracted				
focused				
bored				
ideas				
dissociated				
aware				

Weather:

Meds		Energy Levels	
am		5 - high	
pm		4	
		3	
Hygiene		2	
brush teeth		1 - low	
shower		**Food**	
change clothes			
Intake			
caffeine			
alcohol			
water			
TV			
social media			
time outside		**Creative Space**	
Sleep Hours			
dreamy			
restless			
light			
deep			
terror			

Notes - Wins

Day: Date: /   /20

Physical	Morn	After	Eve	12am+
headache				
nausea				
pain				
menstrual				
fatigue				

Emotional	Morn	After	Eve	12am+
anxious				
calm				
panic				
irritable				
overwhelmed				
depressed				
manic				
excited				
content				

Mental	Morn	After	Eve	12am+
hopeless				
hopeful				
distracted				
focused				
bored				
ideas				
dissociated				
aware				

Weather:

Meds		Energy Levels	
am		5 - high	
pm		4	
		3	
Hygiene		2	
brush teeth		1 - low	
shower			
change clothes		**Food**	
Intake			
caffeine			
alcohol			
water			
TV			
social media			
time outside		**Creative Space**	
Sleep Hours			
dreamy			
restless			
light			
deep			
terror			

Notes - Wins

Notes

Creative Space

Day: Date: /   /20

Physical	Morn	After	Eve	12am+
headache				
nausea				
pain				
menstrual				
fatigue				
Emotional	Morn	After	Eve	12am+
anxious				
calm				
panic				
irritable				
overwhelmed				
depressed				
manic				
excited				
content				
Mental	Morn	After	Eve	12am+
hopeless				
hopeful				
distracted				
focused				
bored				
ideas				
dissociated				
aware				

Weather:

Meds		Energy Levels	
am		5 - high	
pm		4	
		3	
Hygiene		2	
brush teeth		1 - low	
shower			
change clothes		**Food**	
Intake			
caffeine			
alcohol			
water			
TV			
social media			
time outside		**Creative Space**	
Sleep Hours			
dreamy			
restless			
light			
deep			
terror			

Notes - Wins

Day: Date: / /20

Physical	Morn	After	Eve	12am+
headache				
nausea				
pain				
menstrual				
fatigue				

Emotional	Morn	After	Eve	12am+
anxious				
calm				
panic				
irritable				
overwhelmed				
depressed				
manic				
excited				
content				

Mental	Morn	After	Eve	12am+
hopeless				
hopeful				
distracted				
focused				
bored				
ideas				
dissociated				
aware				

Weather:

Meds		Energy Levels	
am		5 - high	
pm		4	
		3	
Hygiene		2	
brush teeth		1 - low	
shower			
change clothes		**Food**	
Intake			
caffeine			
alcohol			
water			
TV			
social media			
time outside		**Creative Space**	
Sleep Hours			
dreamy			
restless			
light			
deep			
terror			

Notes - Wins

Day: Date: /   /20

Physical	Morn	After	Eve	12am+
headache				
nausea				
pain				
menstrual				
fatigue				

Emotional	Morn	After	Eve	12am+
anxious				
calm				
panic				
irritable				
overwhelmed				
depressed				
manic				
excited				
content				

Mental	Morn	After	Eve	12am+
hopeless				
hopeful				
distracted				
focused				
bored				
ideas				
dissociated				
aware				

Weather:

Meds		Energy Levels	
am		5 - high	
pm		4	
		3	
Hygiene		2	
brush teeth		1 - low	
shower			
change clothes		**Food**	
Intake			
caffeine			
alcohol			
water			
TV			
social media			
time outside		**Creative Space**	
Sleep Hours			
dreamy			
restless			
light			
deep			
terror			

Notes - Wins

Day: Date: /   /20

Physical	Morn	After	Eve	12am+
headache				
nausea				
pain				
menstrual				
fatigue				

Emotional	Morn	After	Eve	12am+
anxious				
calm				
panic				
irritable				
overwhelmed				
depressed				
manic				
excited				
content				

Mental	Morn	After	Eve	12am+
hopeless				
hopeful				
distracted				
focused				
bored				
ideas				
dissociated				
aware				

Weather:

Meds		Energy Levels	
am		5 - high	
pm		4	
		3	
Hygiene		2	
brush teeth		1 - low	
shower			
change clothes		**Food**	
Intake			
caffeine			
alcohol			
water			
TV			
social media			
time outside		**Creative Space**	
Sleep Hours			
dreamy			
restless			
light			
deep			
terror			

Notes - Wins

Day: Date: /   /20

Physical	Morn	After	Eve	12am+
headache				
nausea				
pain				
menstrual				
fatigue				

Emotional	Morn	After	Eve	12am+
anxious				
calm				
panic				
irritable				
overwhelmed				
depressed				
manic				
excited				
content				

Mental	Morn	After	Eve	12am+
hopeless				
hopeful				
distracted				
focused				
bored				
ideas				
dissociated				
aware				

Weather:

Meds		Energy Levels	
am		5 - high	
pm		4	
		3	
Hygiene		2	
brush teeth		1 - low	
shower			
change clothes		**Food**	
Intake			
caffeine			
alcohol			
water			
TV			
social media			
time outside		**Creative Space**	
Sleep Hours			
dreamy			
restless			
light			
deep			
terror			

Notes - Wins

Day: Date: /   /20

Physical	Morn	After	Eve	12am+
headache				
nausea				
pain				
menstrual				
fatigue				
Emotional	**Morn**	**After**	**Eve**	**12am+**
anxious				
calm				
panic				
irritable				
overwhelmed				
depressed				
manic				
excited				
content				
Mental	**Morn**	**After**	**Eve**	**12am+**
hopeless				
hopeful				
distracted				
focused				
bored				
ideas				
dissociated				
aware				

Weather:

Meds		Energy Levels	
am		5 - high	
pm		4	
		3	
Hygiene		2	
brush teeth		1 - low	
shower			
change clothes		**Food**	
Intake			
caffeine			
alcohol			
water			
TV			
social media			
time outside		**Creative Space**	
Sleep Hours			
dreamy			
restless			
light			
deep			
terror			

Notes - Wins

Day: Date: /   /20

Physical	Morn	After	Eve	12am+
headache				
nausea				
pain				
menstrual				
fatigue				
Emotional	**Morn**	**After**	**Eve**	**12am+**
anxious				
calm				
panic				
irritable				
overwhelmed				
depressed				
manic				
excited				
content				
Mental	**Morn**	**After**	**Eve**	**12am+**
hopeless				
hopeful				
distracted				
focused				
bored				
ideas				
dissociated				
aware				

Weather:

Meds		Energy Levels	
am		5 - high	
pm		4	
		3	
Hygiene		2	
brush teeth		1 - low	
shower			
change clothes		**Food**	
Intake			
caffeine			
alcohol			
water			
TV			
social media			
time outside		**Creative Space**	
Sleep Hours			
dreamy			
restless			
light			
deep			
terror			

Notes - Wins

Notes

Day: Date: /   /20

Physical	Morn	After	Eve	12am+
headache				
nausea				
pain				
menstrual				
fatigue				

Emotional	Morn	After	Eve	12am+
anxious				
calm				
panic				
irritable				
overwhelmed				
depressed				
manic				
excited				
content				

Mental	Morn	After	Eve	12am+
hopeless				
hopeful				
distracted				
focused				
bored				
ideas				
dissociated				
aware				

Weather:

Meds		Energy Levels	
am		5 - high	
pm		4	
		3	
Hygiene		2	
brush teeth		1 - low	
shower			
change clothes		**Food**	
Intake			
caffeine			
alcohol			
water			
TV			
social media			
time outside		**Creative Space**	
Sleep Hours			
dreamy			
restless			
light			
deep			
terror			

Notes - Wins

Day: Date: /   /20

Physical	Morn	After	Eve	12am+
headache				
nausea				
pain				
menstrual				
fatigue				

Emotional	Morn	After	Eve	12am+
anxious				
calm				
panic				
irritable				
overwhelmed				
depressed				
manic				
excited				
content				

Mental	Morn	After	Eve	12am+
hopeless				
hopeful				
distracted				
focused				
bored				
ideas				
dissociated				
aware				

Weather:

Meds		Energy Levels	
am		5 - high	
pm		4	
		3	
Hygiene		2	
brush teeth		1 - low	
shower			
change clothes		**Food**	
Intake			
caffeine			
alcohol			
water			
TV			
social media			
time outside		**Creative Space**	
Sleep Hours			
dreamy			
restless			
light			
deep			
terror			

Notes - Wins

Day: Date: /   /20

Physical	Morn	After	Eve	12am+
headache				
nausea				
pain				
menstrual				
fatigue				

Emotional	Morn	After	Eve	12am+
anxious				
calm				
panic				
irritable				
overwhelmed				
depressed				
manic				
excited				
content				

Mental	Morn	After	Eve	12am+
hopeless				
hopeful				
distracted				
focused				
bored				
ideas				
dissociated				
aware				

Weather:

Meds		Energy Levels	
am		5 - high	
pm		4	
		3	
Hygiene		2	
brush teeth		1 - low	
shower		**Food**	
change clothes			
Intake			
caffeine			
alcohol			
water			
TV			
social media			
time outside		**Creative Space**	
Sleep Hours			
dreamy			
restless			
light			
deep			
terror			

Notes - Wins

Day: Date: /   /20

Physical	Morn	After	Eve	12am+
headache				
nausea				
pain				
menstrual				
fatigue				

Emotional	Morn	After	Eve	12am+
anxious				
calm				
panic				
irritable				
overwhelmed				
depressed				
manic				
excited				
content				

Mental	Morn	After	Eve	12am+
hopeless				
hopeful				
distracted				
focused				
bored				
ideas				
dissociated				
aware				

Weather:

Meds		Energy Levels	
am		5 - high	
pm		4	
		3	
Hygiene		2	
brush teeth		1 - low	
shower			
change clothes		**Food**	
Intake			
caffeine			
alcohol			
water			
TV			
social media			
time outside		**Creative Space**	
Sleep Hours			
dreamy			
restless			
light			
deep			
terror			

Notes - Wins

Day:　　　　　　　　　　　Date:　　/　　/20

Physical	Morn	After	Eve	12am+
headache				
nausea				
pain				
menstrual				
fatigue				

Emotional	Morn	After	Eve	12am+
anxious				
calm				
panic				
irritable				
overwhelmed				
depressed				
manic				
excited				
content				

Mental	Morn	After	Eve	12am+
hopeless				
hopeful				
distracted				
focused				
bored				
ideas				
dissociated				
aware				

Weather:

Meds		Energy Levels	
am		5 - high	
pm		4	
		3	
Hygiene		2	
brush teeth		1 - low	
shower			
change clothes		**Food**	
Intake			
caffeine			
alcohol			
water			
TV			
social media			
time outside		**Creative Space**	
Sleep Hours			
dreamy			
restless			
light			
deep			
terror			

Notes - Wins

Day: Date: /   /20

Physical	Morn	After	Eve	12am+
headache				
nausea				
pain				
menstrual				
fatigue				

Emotional	Morn	After	Eve	12am+
anxious				
calm				
panic				
irritable				
overwhelmed				
depressed				
manic				
excited				
content				

Mental	Morn	After	Eve	12am+
hopeless				
hopeful				
distracted				
focused				
bored				
ideas				
dissociated				
aware				

Weather:

Meds		Energy Levels	
am		5 - high	
pm		4	
		3	
Hygiene		2	
brush teeth		1 - low	
shower			
change clothes		**Food**	
Intake			
caffeine			
alcohol			
water			
TV			
social media			
time outside		**Creative Space**	
Sleep Hours			
dreamy			
restless			
light			
deep			
terror			

Notes - Wins

Day: Date: /   /20

Physical	Morn	After	Eve	12am+
headache				
nausea				
pain				
menstrual				
fatigue				

Emotional	Morn	After	Eve	12am+
anxious				
calm				
panic				
irritable				
overwhelmed				
depressed				
manic				
excited				
content				

Mental	Morn	After	Eve	12am+
hopeless				
hopeful				
distracted				
focused				
bored				
ideas				
dissociated				
aware				

Weather:

Meds		Energy Levels	
am		5 - high	
pm		4	
		3	
Hygiene		2	
brush teeth		1 - low	
shower			
change clothes		**Food**	
Intake			
caffeine			
alcohol			
water			
TV			
social media			
time outside		**Creative Space**	
Sleep Hours			
dreamy			
restless			
light			
deep			
terror			

Notes - Wins

Notes

Creative Space

Day: Date: /   /20

Physical	Morn	After	Eve	12am+
headache				
nausea				
pain				
menstrual				
fatigue				

Emotional	Morn	After	Eve	12am+
anxious				
calm				
panic				
irritable				
overwhelmed				
depressed				
manic				
excited				
content				

Mental	Morn	After	Eve	12am+
hopeless				
hopeful				
distracted				
focused				
bored				
ideas				
dissociated				
aware				

Weather:

Meds		Energy Levels	
am		5 - high	
pm		4	
		3	
Hygiene		2	
brush teeth		1 - low	
shower			
change clothes		**Food**	
Intake			
caffeine			
alcohol			
water			
TV			
social media			
time outside		**Creative Space**	
Sleep Hours			
dreamy			
restless			
light			
deep			
terror			

Notes - Wins

Day: Date: /   /20

Physical	Morn	After	Eve	12am+
headache				
nausea				
pain				
menstrual				
fatigue				

Emotional	Morn	After	Eve	12am+
anxious				
calm				
panic				
irritable				
overwhelmed				
depressed				
manic				
excited				
content				

Mental	Morn	After	Eve	12am+
hopeless				
hopeful				
distracted				
focused				
bored				
ideas				
dissociated				
aware				

Weather:

Meds		Energy Levels	
am		5 - high	
pm		4	
		3	
Hygiene		2	
brush teeth		1 - low	
shower			
change clothes		**Food**	
Intake			
caffeine			
alcohol			
water			
TV			
social media			
time outside		**Creative Space**	
Sleep Hours			
dreamy			
restless			
light			
deep			
terror			

Notes - Wins

Day: Date: /   /20

Physical	Morn	After	Eve	12am+
headache				
nausea				
pain				
menstrual				
fatigue				

Emotional	Morn	After	Eve	12am+
anxious				
calm				
panic				
irritable				
overwhelmed				
depressed				
manic				
excited				
content				

Mental	Morn	After	Eve	12am+
hopeless				
hopeful				
distracted				
focused				
bored				
ideas				
dissociated				
aware				

Weather:

Meds		Energy Levels	
am		5 - high	
pm		4	
		3	
Hygiene		2	
brush teeth		1 - low	
shower			
change clothes		**Food**	
Intake			
caffeine			
alcohol			
water			
TV			
social media			
time outside		**Creative Space**	
Sleep Hours			
dreamy			
restless			
light			
deep			
terror			

Notes - Wins

Day: Date: / /20

Physical	Morn	After	Eve	12am+
headache				
nausea				
pain				
menstrual				
fatigue				

Emotional	Morn	After	Eve	12am+
anxious				
calm				
panic				
irritable				
overwhelmed				
depressed				
manic				
excited				
content				

Mental	Morn	After	Eve	12am+
hopeless				
hopeful				
distracted				
focused				
bored				
ideas				
dissociated				
aware				

Weather:

Meds		Energy Levels	
am		5 - high	
pm		4	
		3	
Hygiene		2	
brush teeth		1 - low	
shower			
change clothes		**Food**	
Intake			
caffeine			
alcohol			
water			
TV			
social media			
time outside		**Creative Space**	
Sleep Hours			
dreamy			
restless			
light			
deep			
terror			

Notes - Wins

Day: Date: /   /20

Physical	Morn	After	Eve	12am+
headache				
nausea				
pain				
menstrual				
fatigue				

Emotional	Morn	After	Eve	12am+
anxious				
calm				
panic				
irritable				
overwhelmed				
depressed				
manic				
excited				
content				

Mental	Morn	After	Eve	12am+
hopeless				
hopeful				
distracted				
focused				
bored				
ideas				
dissociated				
aware				

Weather:

Meds		Energy Levels	
am		5 - high	
pm		4	
		3	
Hygiene		2	
brush teeth		1 - low	
shower			
change clothes		**Food**	
Intake			
caffeine			
alcohol			
water			
TV			
social media			
time outside		**Creative Space**	
Sleep Hours			
dreamy			
restless			
light			
deep			
terror			

Notes - Wins

Day: Date: /   /20

Physical	Morn	After	Eve	12am+
headache				
nausea				
pain				
menstrual				
fatigue				

Emotional	Morn	After	Eve	12am+
anxious				
calm				
panic				
irritable				
overwhelmed				
depressed				
manic				
excited				
content				

Mental	Morn	After	Eve	12am+
hopeless				
hopeful				
distracted				
focused				
bored				
ideas				
dissociated				
aware				

Weather:

Meds		Energy Levels	
am		5 - high	
pm		4	
		3	
Hygiene		2	
brush teeth		1 - low	
shower			
change clothes		**Food**	
Intake			
caffeine			
alcohol			
water			
TV			
social media			
time outside		**Creative Space**	
Sleep Hours			
dreamy			
restless			
light			
deep			
terror			

Notes - Wins

Day: Date: /   /20

Physical	Morn	After	Eve	12am+
headache				
nausea				
pain				
menstrual				
fatigue				

Emotional	Morn	After	Eve	12am+
anxious				
calm				
panic				
irritable				
overwhelmed				
depressed				
manic				
excited				
content				

Mental	Morn	After	Eve	12am+
hopeless				
hopeful				
distracted				
focused				
bored				
ideas				
dissociated				
aware				

Weather:

Meds		Energy Levels	
am		5 - high	
pm		4	
		3	
Hygiene		2	
brush teeth		1 - low	
shower			
change clothes		**Food**	
Intake			
caffeine			
alcohol			
water			
TV			
social media			
time outside		**Creative Space**	
Sleep Hours			
dreamy			
restless			
light			
deep			
terror			

Notes - Wins

Notes

Creative Space

Day: Date: /   /20

Physical	Morn	After	Eve	12am+
headache				
nausea				
pain				
menstrual				
fatigue				

Emotional	Morn	After	Eve	12am+
anxious				
calm				
panic				
irritable				
overwhelmed				
depressed				
manic				
excited				
content				

Mental	Morn	After	Eve	12am+
hopeless				
hopeful				
distracted				
focused				
bored				
ideas				
dissociated				
aware				

Weather:

Meds		Energy Levels	
am		5 - high	
pm		4	
		3	
Hygiene		2	
brush teeth		1 - low	
shower			
change clothes		**Food**	
Intake			
caffeine			
alcohol			
water			
TV			
social media			
time outside		**Creative Space**	
Sleep Hours			
dreamy			
restless			
light			
deep			
terror			

Notes - Wins

Day: Date: /   /20

Physical	Morn	After	Eve	12am+
headache				
nausea				
pain				
menstrual				
fatigue				

Emotional	Morn	After	Eve	12am+
anxious				
calm				
panic				
irritable				
overwhelmed				
depressed				
manic				
excited				
content				

Mental	Morn	After	Eve	12am+
hopeless				
hopeful				
distracted				
focused				
bored				
ideas				
dissociated				
aware				

Weather:

Meds		Energy Levels	
am		5 - high	
pm		4	
		3	
Hygiene		2	
brush teeth		1 - low	
shower			
change clothes		**Food**	
Intake			
caffeine			
alcohol			
water			
TV			
social media			
time outside		**Creative Space**	
Sleep Hours			
dreamy			
restless			
light			
deep			
terror			

Notes - Wins

Day: Date: /   /20

Physical	Morn	After	Eve	12am+
headache				
nausea				
pain				
menstrual				
fatigue				

Emotional	Morn	After	Eve	12am+
anxious				
calm				
panic				
irritable				
overwhelmed				
depressed				
manic				
excited				
content				

Mental	Morn	After	Eve	12am+
hopeless				
hopeful				
distracted				
focused				
bored				
ideas				
dissociated				
aware				

Weather:

Meds		Energy Levels	
am		5 - high	
pm		4	
		3	
Hygiene		2	
brush teeth		1 - low	
shower			
change clothes		**Food**	
Intake			
caffeine			
alcohol			
water			
TV			
social media			
time outside		**Creative Space**	
Sleep Hours			
dreamy			
restless			
light			
deep			
terror			

Notes - Wins

Day: Date: /   /20

Physical	Morn	After	Eve	12am+
headache				
nausea				
pain				
menstrual				
fatigue				

Emotional	Morn	After	Eve	12am+
anxious				
calm				
panic				
irritable				
overwhelmed				
depressed				
manic				
excited				
content				

Mental	Morn	After	Eve	12am+
hopeless				
hopeful				
distracted				
focused				
bored				
ideas				
dissociated				
aware				

Weather:

Meds		Energy Levels	
am		5 - high	
pm		4	
		3	
Hygiene		2	
brush teeth		1 - low	
shower			
change clothes		**Food**	
Intake			
caffeine			
alcohol			
water			
TV			
social media			
time outside		**Creative Space**	
Sleep Hours			
dreamy			
restless			
light			
deep			
terror			

Notes - Wins

Day: Date: /   /20

Physical	Morn	After	Eve	12am+
headache				
nausea				
pain				
menstrual				
fatigue				

Emotional	Morn	After	Eve	12am+
anxious				
calm				
panic				
irritable				
overwhelmed				
depressed				
manic				
excited				
content				

Mental	Morn	After	Eve	12am+
hopeless				
hopeful				
distracted				
focused				
bored				
ideas				
dissociated				
aware				

Weather:

Meds		Energy Levels	
am		5 - high	
pm		4	
		3	
Hygiene		2	
brush teeth		1 - low	
shower			
change clothes		**Food**	
Intake			
caffeine			
alcohol			
water			
TV			
social media			
time outside		**Creative Space**	
Sleep Hours			
dreamy			
restless			
light			
deep			
terror			

Notes - Wins

Day: Date: /   /20

Physical	Morn	After	Eve	12am+
headache				
nausea				
pain				
menstrual				
fatigue				

Emotional	Morn	After	Eve	12am+
anxious				
calm				
panic				
irritable				
overwhelmed				
depressed				
manic				
excited				
content				

Mental	Morn	After	Eve	12am+
hopeless				
hopeful				
distracted				
focused				
bored				
ideas				
dissociated				
aware				

Weather:

Meds		Energy Levels	
am		5 - high	
pm		4	
		3	
Hygiene		2	
brush teeth		1 - low	
shower			
change clothes		**Food**	
Intake			
caffeine			
alcohol			
water			
TV			
social media			
time outside		**Creative Space**	
Sleep Hours			
dreamy			
restless			
light			
deep			
terror			

Notes - Wins

Day: Date: /   /20

Physical	Morn	After	Eve	12am+
headache				
nausea				
pain				
menstrual				
fatigue				
Emotional	**Morn**	**After**	**Eve**	**12am+**
anxious				
calm				
panic				
irritable				
overwhelmed				
depressed				
manic				
excited				
content				
Mental	**Morn**	**After**	**Eve**	**12am+**
hopeless				
hopeful				
distracted				
focused				
bored				
ideas				
dissociated				
aware				

Weather:

Meds		Energy Levels	
am		5 - high	
pm		4	
		3	
Hygiene		2	
brush teeth		1 - low	
shower			
change clothes		**Food**	
Intake			
caffeine			
alcohol			
water			
TV			
social media			
time outside		**Creative Space**	
Sleep Hours			
dreamy			
restless			
light			
deep			
terror			

Notes - Wins

Notes

Day: Date: / /20

Physical	Morn	After	Eve	12am+
headache				
nausea				
pain				
menstrual				
fatigue				

Emotional	Morn	After	Eve	12am+
anxious				
calm				
panic				
irritable				
overwhelmed				
depressed				
manic				
excited				
content				

Mental	Morn	After	Eve	12am+
hopeless				
hopeful				
distracted				
focused				
bored				
ideas				
dissociated				
aware				

Weather:

Meds		Energy Levels	
am		5 - high	
pm		4	
		3	
Hygiene		2	
brush teeth		1 - low	
shower			
change clothes		**Food**	
Intake			
caffeine			
alcohol			
water			
TV			
social media			
time outside		**Creative Space**	
Sleep Hours			
dreamy			
restless			
light			
deep			
terror			

Notes - Wins

Day: Date: /   /20

Physical	Morn	After	Eve	12am+
headache				
nausea				
pain				
menstrual				
fatigue				

Emotional	Morn	After	Eve	12am+
anxious				
calm				
panic				
irritable				
overwhelmed				
depressed				
manic				
excited				
content				

Mental	Morn	After	Eve	12am+
hopeless				
hopeful				
distracted				
focused				
bored				
ideas				
dissociated				
aware				

Weather:

Meds		Energy Levels	
am		5 - high	
pm		4	
		3	
Hygiene		2	
brush teeth		1 - low	
shower			
change clothes		**Food**	
Intake			
caffeine			
alcohol			
water			
TV			
social media			
time outside		**Creative Space**	
Sleep Hours			
dreamy			
restless			
light			
deep			
terror			

Notes - Wins

Day: Date: /   /20

Physical	Morn	After	Eve	12am+
headache				
nausea				
pain				
menstrual				
fatigue				

Emotional	Morn	After	Eve	12am+
anxious				
calm				
panic				
irritable				
overwhelmed				
depressed				
manic				
excited				
content				

Mental	Morn	After	Eve	12am+
hopeless				
hopeful				
distracted				
focused				
bored				
ideas				
dissociated				
aware				

Weather:

Meds		Energy Levels	
am		5 - high	
pm		4	
		3	
Hygiene		2	
brush teeth		1 - low	
shower			
change clothes		**Food**	
Intake			
caffeine			
alcohol			
water			
TV			
social media			
time outside		**Creative Space**	
Sleep Hours			
dreamy			
restless			
light			
deep			
terror			

Notes - Wins

Day: Date: /   /20

Physical	Morn	After	Eve	12am+
headache				
nausea				
pain				
menstrual				
fatigue				

Emotional	Morn	After	Eve	12am+
anxious				
calm				
panic				
irritable				
overwhelmed				
depressed				
manic				
excited				
content				

Mental	Morn	After	Eve	12am+
hopeless				
hopeful				
distracted				
focused				
bored				
ideas				
dissociated				
aware				

Weather:

Meds		Energy Levels	
am		5 - high	
pm		4	
		3	
Hygiene		2	
brush teeth		1 - low	
shower			
change clothes		**Food**	
Intake			
caffeine			
alcohol			
water			
TV			
social media			
time outside		**Creative Space**	
Sleep Hours			
dreamy			
restless			
light			
deep			
terror			

Notes - Wins

Day: Date: /   /20

Physical	Morn	After	Eve	12am+
headache				
nausea				
pain				
menstrual				
fatigue				

Emotional	Morn	After	Eve	12am+
anxious				
calm				
panic				
irritable				
overwhelmed				
depressed				
manic				
excited				
content				

Mental	Morn	After	Eve	12am+
hopeless				
hopeful				
distracted				
focused				
bored				
ideas				
dissociated				
aware				

Weather:

Meds		Energy Levels	
am		5 - high	
pm		4	
		3	
Hygiene		2	
brush teeth		1 - low	
shower			
change clothes		**Food**	
Intake			
caffeine			
alcohol			
water			
TV			
social media			
time outside		**Creative Space**	
Sleep Hours			
dreamy			
restless			
light			
deep			
terror			

Notes - Wins

Day: Date: /   /20

Physical	Morn	After	Eve	12am+
headache				
nausea				
pain				
menstrual				
fatigue				

Emotional	Morn	After	Eve	12am+
anxious				
calm				
panic				
irritable				
overwhelmed				
depressed				
manic				
excited				
content				

Mental	Morn	After	Eve	12am+
hopeless				
hopeful				
distracted				
focused				
bored				
ideas				
dissociated				
aware				

Weather:

Meds		Energy Levels	
am		5 - high	
pm		4	
		3	
Hygiene		2	
brush teeth		1 - low	
shower			
change clothes		**Food**	
Intake			
caffeine			
alcohol			
water			
TV			
social media			
time outside		**Creative Space**	
Sleep Hours			
dreamy			
restless			
light			
deep			
terror			

Notes - Wins

Day: Date: / /20

Physical	Morn	After	Eve	12am+
headache				
nausea				
pain				
menstrual				
fatigue				

Emotional	Morn	After	Eve	12am+
anxious				
calm				
panic				
irritable				
overwhelmed				
depressed				
manic				
excited				
content				

Mental	Morn	After	Eve	12am+
hopeless				
hopeful				
distracted				
focused				
bored				
ideas				
dissociated				
aware				

Weather:

Meds		Energy Levels	
am		5 - high	
pm		4	
		3	
Hygiene		2	
brush teeth		1 - low	
shower			
change clothes		**Food**	
Intake			
caffeine			
alcohol			
water			
TV			
social media		**Creative Space**	
time outside			
Sleep Hours			
dreamy			
restless			
light			
deep			
terror			

Notes - Wins

Notes